I0439419

TABLE OF CONTENTS

Anti Aging Techniques EXPOSED Vol 3
Unlock the Mysteries of Feeling Young
©Copyright 2013 by Dr. Noah Pranksky

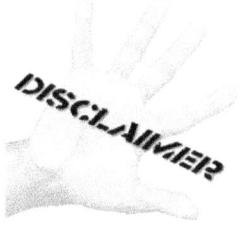

DISCLAIMER AND TERMS OF USE AGREEMENT:

(Please Read This Before Using This Book)

This information is for educational and informational purposes only. The content is not intended to be a substitute for any professional advice, diagnosis, or treatment.

The authors and publisher of this book and the accompanying materials have used their best efforts in preparing this book.

The authors and publisher make no representation or warranties with respect to the accuracy, applicability, fitness, or completeness of the contents of this book. The information contained in this book is strictly for educational purposes. Therefore, if you wish to apply

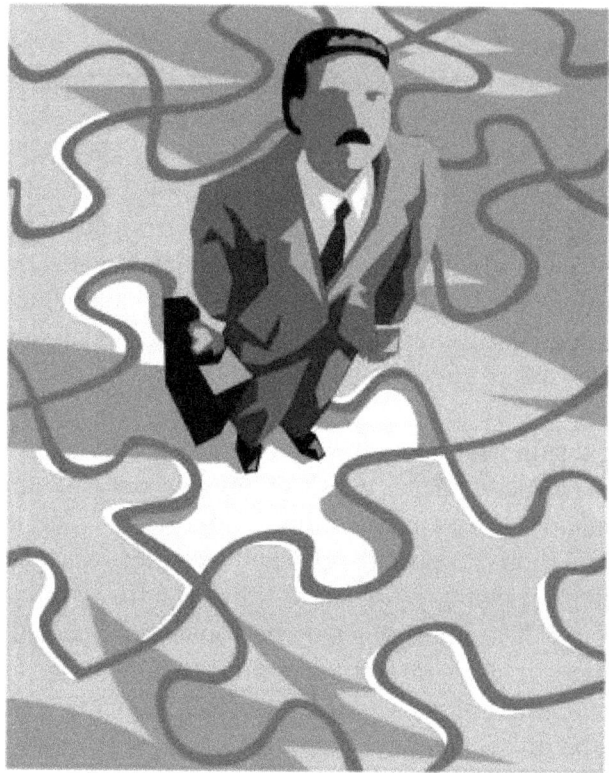

In Volume 2, we touched briefly on how the mind affects the body and vice versa. All the parts are connected so I want to begin by delving deeper into the concept of The Complete Person.

Physiologically speaking, the body operates around the central nervous system; made up of two sub-systems called the somatic nervous system (this is the system that gives you volitional control of your muscles and skeletal

4

movements) and the autonomic nervous system (this is the system, which regulates our glands and correlates with our emotions).

The central nervous system includes the brain, and spinal cord. The autonomic nervous system tells the brain, which stimuli have been received; the brain responds based upon how it has been programmed. Since an individual is the sum total of his/her experiences, the brain is programmed based on these experiences, as well as perceived experience.

The brain IS NOT the mind!

The mind resides in the brain but they are two separate and distinct entities. The best way to describe all of the "parts," using computer terminology, is the autonomic nervous system is the software, the brain is the hardware, and the mind is the hard drive.

You must never forget the "Complete Person" concept, as you attempt to practice proper healthy protocols and the practice of healthy protocols is a big part of staying young and retarding the effects of aging...

A human body is made up of atoms, cells, chemicals, minerals, and various structures. The body has numerous different systems, such as digestion, circulation, respiration, lymphatic, immune, and nervous, to name but a few, and these each have unique operations which involve utilizing material from the environment to keep the body going.

The body is a tremendously complex biological mechanism. There is no man-made thing anywhere that comes even slightly close to it in terms of the sheer amount of systems, relationships of systems, and complexity.

Specific body functions monitor and handle sugar levels, electrolyte relations, mineral levels and ratios, blood oxygen levels, cellular toxicity, and *thousands* of other things known not yet discovered or known.

Apparently the body keeps itself running and functioning just fine if left to itself and allowed to heal itself. This FACT is one thing you will never hear come out of a doctor's mouth that the body's own inherent intelligence operates continually, 24 hours a day, to keep it going, and to keep it going at an optimum level. *It*, whatever "it" is, "knows" what to do at the smallest cellular level right on up to the largest interactive whole body level.

Anyone who cares to observe and learn about the various body functions will be truly amazed at what the physical body does all by itself. The body ingests, assimilates, organizes and utilizes various chemicals, minerals, vitamins, and enzymes as the raw material to keep itself going. Thousands upon thousands of chemical reactions at a cellular and organ level occur in your body each and every second! So, if the chemicals aren't adequately supplied, or if certain of the body's monitoring and organizing functions become impaired due to a past failure to obtain the needed chemicals, it can't remain "healthy".

The body needs raw materials such as minerals, water, vitamins, and various chemicals, which it largely gets through food (i.e. nutrition), but also from the air and water. These keep the body machine running and also keep it in good "mechanical" shape. This is common sense, although apparently not to the modern western-oriented medical doctor.

And so many modern doctors pooh-pooh nutritional approaches to health. They sometimes use the notion of the "starry eyed, hippie, health food fanatic" and attempt to attach it to the entire nutritional approach with the purpose of diminishing the public's perception of it as valid and useful.

A generalized caricature of the health-food fanatic is often attached to the various subjects of alternative medicine and used to prevent an accurate perception and understanding of these subjects. Sadly, these tactics work far too often. Too many people accept without question the conceptual associations given to them by others, no matter how untrue or inaccurate these might be.

The modern medical doctors have nothing to do with "creating health". They are only concerned with eradicating or destroying disease, and the removing of disease (which is usually only a group of *symptoms* of some underlying and unrecognized physical problem) is a very incomplete and one-sided approach to the complete subject called "health".

It's not that modern medical techniques don't have their place, they do, but their approach is only an isolated part of a much larger picture. The picture they present of themselves as being the *whole picture* is simply incorrect, and has devastating effects on people, the quality of life and society.

Chapter 1 - How to Reduce Stress Level

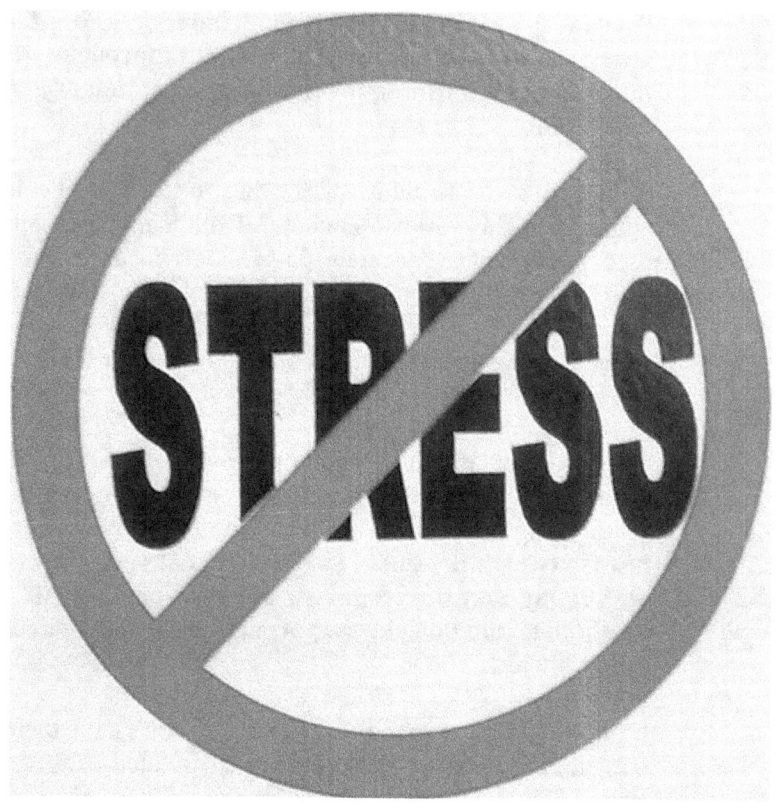

What I am about to introduce to you is a subject that can be easily misunderstood. And I will show you just how easy things can be misunderstood.

I am not attempting to start a cult; I am not asking anyone to drink the Kool-Aid, but I am asking you to open your minds and see things from a different perspective especially when it pertains to cause and effect visa vie anti aging...

I am also not asking people to take their medical needs into their own hands and ignore competent medical advice. I firmly believe that people have definitive medical needs that a medical professional can and should address.

Most people will experience anxiety in their lifetime. Without understanding truly what anxiety and stress really are, people are suffering from problems they know little about. And since the mind affects the body and vice versa, stress and anxiety definitely affects the aging process!

So first, let's define anxiety. Anxiety is a general term used for nervousness, fear, apprehension or worry associated with uncertain outcomes. In other words, anxiety is fear over what MAY happen either real or perceived. Examples are panic disorders, OCD, PTSD, phobias, etc.

Here are some eye-opening statistics:

- One out of seven Americans, ages 18 and above, is said to suffer from an anxiety disorder. This is close to 42-million Americans or almost 19% of our population.

- Anxiety disorders are the number 1 mental health problem among women and the number 2 mental health problem among men.

- Women are twice as likely to suffer from anxiety as men.

Is there a reasonable solution? Yes, however, as I have said in the past, as a whole people like a diagnosis more than they like the solution. Because a diagnosis allows us to make excuses for what our lives have become and a solution challenges us to take steps for what our lives could be. In other words, it allows us to become victims of something other than ourselves and today our country is made up almost exclusively of victims.

So is the solution as simple as focus? Is what our minds focus on the underlying cause of anxiety and stress? Let's see...

There are thousands of experts and just as many critics involved in the field of anxiety and stress. But all of them generally agree on four areas of viewpoint when it comes to anxiety and stress:

- Rooting around in your past experiences, primarily in your childhood, will reveal areas of problems and tension that lead to the anxiety you are suffering from today. And for $120 per hour, several times per week, for a number of years, they will be happy to play 20-questions with you.

- Others claim that the problem is environmental. If you remove the person from that particular environment then the problem is solved.

- Some even suggest that the problem can be traced back to a chemical imbalance in the brain causing the neurons to misfire and hence...anxiety.

- People focus on the wrong thoughts rather than thinking through positive thoughts. If you replace the negative with the positive than the power of positive thinking is enough to solve the problem.

"Why is all of this happening now?"

In other words, is this a generational issue, is this an American issue, and is this a human issue? Let's pull back for a moment and frame this in a context that is much bigger.

Is this a human problem or is this a relatively new problem? If it is a human problem, then it should be seen in every generation, in every people group worldwide.

My take on this is simple: anxiety here in America is about a fifty year phenomena within this culture and not humanity as a whole. From 1910 to 1950 our grandparents and parents experience two world wars and the Great Depression. If any one group had a better claim to depression, anxiety and stress it would be our parents and grandparents. They should have been the most messed up generation closest to our generation. But they came home and started businesses, saved money, put their kids through college, and built America into the world power it is today. And they did all this before prescription drugs dealt with the subject of anxiety and stress!

Nobody told them to go back and look into their childhood to find their issues. So once again is this a human problem or generational problem?

How does money factor in this? On third...ONE THIRD...of the $148 billion dollars spent annually on mental health is eaten up dealing with anxiety disorders. So, before we accept all of the current research on anxiety disorders, we need to go back and ask who paid for this research.

Bottom line: ANXIETY IS BIG BUSINESS AND SOMEONE IS GETTING PAID AND SOMEONE IS GETTING PAID REAL WELL!

And I am not alone in my scepticism either. There are thousands of doctors sounding the alarm saying watch out because the medication given to people to treat anxiety disorders is doing irreparable harm

Dr. Peter Breggin in his book "Brain Disabling Treatments in Psychiatry" said, "At present, there are no known bio-chemical imbalances in the brain of typical psychiatric patients until they are given psychiatric drugs."

Dr. Eric Nestler of Yale University School of Medicine, "Psychiatric drugs are like sledgehammers; they profoundly alter many of the pathways in our brain."

Dr. Lorrin Koran states, "A physical disease that is incorrectly diagnosed as a mental disorder can lead to a lifetime on psychotropic drugs, loss of productivity, physical and social deterioration and shattered dreams."

Dr. David Kaiser points out, "Patients have been diagnosed with chemical imbalances despite the fact that no test exists to support such a claim."
Now let's delve deeper into the subject and learn about the core foundation of what doctors use to treat anxiety disorders.

The best way to alleviate stress is to first understand what stress is and what is not stress. The next step is to remove the "triggers' to your stress or alleviate their effects.

Today, there are a good many things to be stressful about – the economy, children, health, taxes but you can't remove these "triggers" from your life but you can move to alleviate their effects in your life. You are accountable to YOU!

Self-medicating yourself away from your problems is not the answer. Drugs, alcohol, smoking and binge eating only cause more harm. You must learn to cope with what you have and look for solutions that will improve your life. This will guarantee the retardation of the aging process.

Chapter 2 - Supplement Your Genes

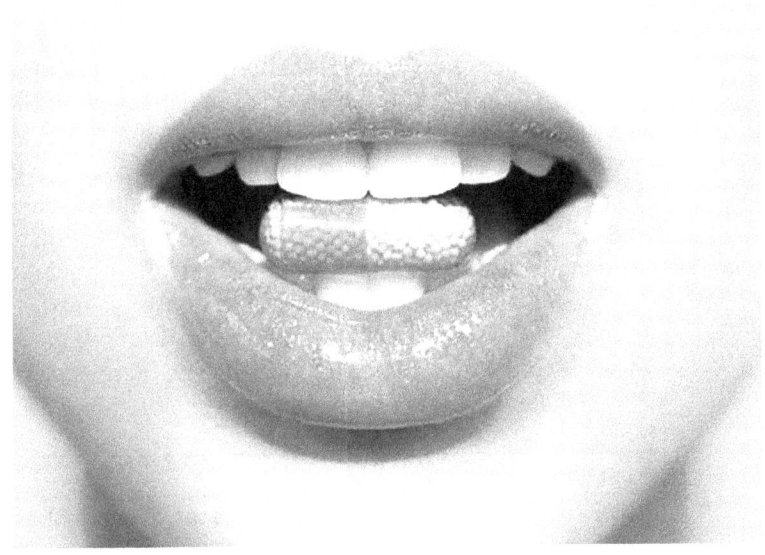

Do You Really Need All Those Supplements?

In answering a question as complicated and important as this one, we must look to scientific fact rather than the host of opinions that bombard the American consumer. One fact is this: the optimum daily amounts of vitamins and minerals are far larger than the amounts that can be obtained in food. This is because of present day farming techniques and an increase in the amount of processed food Americans ingest daily. The quality has decreased and Americans have increased the quantity of consumption. Poor food and poor eating habits require us to use supplements.

Choosing a Responsibly Made Vitamin

Vitamins either enable biochemical reactions in the body to take place more effectively, or they prevent specific substances from interfering with the biochemical reactions. **Why do I need to take vitamins?** If our soil was not depleted and we did not use pesticides and herbicides on our crops, which greatly reduce the bioavailability of the nutrients to be metabolized, and we ate fruits and vegetables within 6-days of harvesting, and we didn't heat process our food, and add preservatives to them-we wouldn't need to take vitamins. **What should I look for in a vitamin?** Consumers need to be well informed when making the decision to ingest any substance. In considering a supplement, the guidelines for determining if a supplement is responsibly made should include: Heat Processing and Tableting, Iron -Why it should NOT be present, Vitamin-C, Vitamin-D, Beta Carotene, B-Complexes, Chelation and Minerals, Timed-Released, and Synergists.

Heat Processing and Tableting

Look for a supplement that is not heat processed. Tablets are heat processed and capsules are not. Capsules cost the manufacturer more, so most manufacturers tend to use the tableting method. Capsules or pure powders deliver the highest potency. Also, fillers and binders are used to make a tablet hold together, and these binders may cause allergic reactions in some people. Many people think they are allergic to vitamins when they are really only allergic to the binder or filler. Also, tableting may cause extrusion of oil-soluble vitamins from the formulation. For example, a tablet press compresses at 5000 psi which can release beadleted oil-soluble Vitamin A from the protective coat. The Vitamin A then degrades rapidly.

Iron – Why it Should NOT be Present

Look for a complete vitamin/mineral supplement that does not contain iron. Studies have shown that "increased body iron stores are associated with an increase risk of cancer": New England Journal of Medicine. This does not refer to iron found in food or the iron found in protein powders, but to supplemental iron. Also, studies indicate that two-in-four hundred Caucasians have Hemochromatosis; an inherited disorder that causes iron overload and the symptoms can be quite severe. Iron deficiencies in males are rare. Some women do have iron deficiencies in which case an increase in dietary intake of iron rich foods may eliminate the problem. If dietary readjustment does not alleviate the deficiency, an iron supplement may be taken once or twice a week until serum iron levels reach the normal range.

Vitamin-C

The data on Vitamin-C is so extensive that it is unnecessary to validate its value. I would not take more than 500 mgs of Vitamin-C per day. **Megadoses are not advisable** (Are we really meant to consume 20-30 oranges a day? Does this make sense to you?). Megadoses of Vitamin-C depress sperm motility and decreases fertility. It also blunts the beneficial effects of chemotherapy treatment for breast cancer. Cancer cells have numerous receptors for Vitamin-C making it act as a growth tonic for cancer cells. Also, its own synergist, the bioflavonoids, should always accompany Vitamin-C. Vitamin-C does not occur in nature without its sisters, rutin and hesperidin-both bioflavonoids, and any well-made vitamin should mimic nature as closely as possible. Note: Smoking depletes almost 50% of the vitamin-C in the body.

Vitamin-D

Vitamin-D is a vitamin, which acts like a hormone and is the only vitamin the human body can manufacture. In its absence, calcium and phosphorus become immobile and leeching of these two minerals becomes inevitable. In addition, as we age, our ability to synthesize Vitamin-D slows to one-half. Though we need Vitamin-D, it is potentially very toxic, so a safe supplement will not contain large amounts of Vitamin-D. We do not recommend taking a Vitamin-D supplement. **If your body is getting the proper amount of essential fatty acids (Omega 3, 6, 9 oils) your body will make a sufficient amount of Vitamin-D.** Most of the Vitamin-D utilized in the body comes from sunlight interacting with the essential fatty acids in the skin. Therefore, supplemental Vitamin-D without the benefit of sunlight is insufficient for total health. Sun exposure (with sunscreen) should include 20-minutes of summer sun exposure and 40-minutes of winter sun exposure. Be advised that an excessive amount of Vitamin-D causes a magnesium deficiency in the body. Furthermore, megadoses of Vitamin-D irritate the lining of blood vessels and are one of the causes of atherosclerosis.

Beta Carotene

Beta Carotene (Pro-Vitamin A or plant derived Vitamin A) is a natural substance found in fruits and vegetables, which, once inside the body, converts to Vitamin A. Vitamin A is crucial in normal cellular control. Since the body must get Vitamin A from outside sources, when the body does not receive an adequate supply of Vitamin A, cell function becomes abnormal, and cell maturation does not take place. Cells deprived of Vitamin A dedifferentiate, and enter a state paralleling cancerous cells. Stress (including both colds and flu) can deplete up to 60% of the Vitamin A in the body. At St. Luke's Medical Center in Chicago, an important study involving beta-carotene and lung cancer was conducted. It involved 2,107 workers at the Western Electric Company in Chicago. Thirty-Three (33) of the men developed lung cancer, all related to cigarette smoking. The rate of cancer was lowest in those people consuming the highest amounts of beta-carotene foods and the highest in the group consuming the least amounts of beta-carotene foods. The actual ratio turned out to be an 8-to-1 difference in risk between the lowest and highest groups. Beta Carotene can actually negate gene mutation, which occurs when the body is exposed to environmental toxins such as cigarette smoke. The incidence of lung cancer in smokers (2 packs a day for 30-years) who consumed diets high in beta-carotene was similar to the incidence of lung cancer in non-smokers. This is phenomenal data evidencing the powerful anti-carcinogenic properties of beta-carotene. Unused Vitamin A is stored in the liver and can be toxic when taken for extended periods at high doses, where as beta-carotene is considered nontoxic at very high doses. A combination of beta-carotene and Vitamin A (in moderate doses) in a supplement is preferable.

B-Complexes

The B-Vitamins include: B-1 (Thiamin), B-2 (Riboflavin), B-5 (pantothenic acid), B-6 (pyridoxine), B-12 (Cobalamin), PABA (para-aminobenzoic acid), folate (folic acid), inositol, biotin and choline. **Because of modern food processing, it is extremely difficult to obtain even the minimum amount of B-Complexes from our food alone.** Current labeling shows the amount of nutrients found in a food before processing, not after. Flour, for example, loses 82% of its B-vitamins in processing, and spaghetti 64%. Even cracked wheat bread has lost 38% of its B-vitamins. A deficiency of just one of the B-vitamins, thiamin causes extreme mood swings due to lack of availability of serotonin, a brain chemical which help regulate emotions. Patients complaining of lethargy, personality changes, and sleep disturbances, lack of appetite, diarrhea, and fevers of unknown origin were studied. These symptoms "would represent a trap for the unwary physician since he would be unable to find any objective physical sign other than variations of normal, which would be easily classed as the effects of a chronic state of anxiety" (American Journal of Clinical Nutrition). When supplemental Thiamin was given, all patients in the study reported a marked symptomatic improvement or a complete loss of all symptoms.

Ingestion of coffee, either regular or decaffeinated, severely depletes Thiamin. Thiamin isn't alone in its ability to affect moods. Niacin depletion causes severe reactions in humans. "If all the niacin were removed from our food, everyone would be psychotic in one year," (Abram Hoffer, MD and psychiatrist). B-vitamins are also catalysts in the burning of carbohydrates and in glucose tolerance. B-vitamins are water-soluble (Oil-soluble vitamins are A, D, E, and K) so taking them in the morning with breakfast and again with lunch will help insure high energy throughout the day. There are many good quality B-complex supplements for women available in health stores. Be sure to read the labels and understand what you are ingesting. Niacin can cause "flushing" in doses over 30-50mgs, so you may wish to take niacin separately and use a supplement with the "non-flushing" form of niacin, "niacinamide". Niacinamide lacks the beneficial vasodialating effects found in niacin, but "flushing" frightens those who do not understand that flushing is beneficial and is often replaced by niacinamide for that reason.

Chelation and Minerals

Without the proper minerals, vitamins cannot be fully utilized. Minerals are the building blocks for body tissue and other body structures. Minerals enable enzymes and hormones, which regulate the metabolism. Also, minerals maximize the efficiency of healthy essential oils containing the all-important essential fatty acids. Minerals are inorganic and are co-enzymes. Our bodies cannot use raw minerals when taken in their inorganic form because they cannot be digested or used. Plants transform minerals from the soil into an organic form that humans can use by eating vegetables as well as eating animals that have eaten plants and have the minerals present in their meat. The minerals in a supplement should be

18

chelated (bound or "hooked up") to another substance such as an amino acid to promote better bioavailability. Most mineral supplements commonly described as "chelated" have an organic molecule like a citrate or gluconate chemically tied to the mineral, which has a very low bioavailability. Since the intestinal wall readily absorbs proteins, avoid the following so-called chelating agents that are not protein based: citrates, sulfates, gluconates, phosphates, etc.). Chelated minerals are less irritating to the gastrointestinal tract compared to some of the salts of these minerals. We waste money on supplements the body cannot use effectively. For example: By swallowing a 200mg pill of calcium less than 14% is used by the body which translates into 28% bio-availability. Take a 500mg pill of calcium and the body uses almost 70%. How effectively a nutritional supplement is absorbed is far more important than how much is taken. For example: the calcium absorption rate for milk is 30%. For ideal mineral absorption, the ration of minerals to amino acid bonding must be in the ratio between 1-unit of mineral to 3-units of amino acid; the weight of the amino acids in the mineral chelate must be very small (150 Daltons), the total molecular weight must be less than 800 Daltons, and the chelate must not ionize in the digestive system. Digestion quickly separates the commonly used chelating mineral salts or complexes from any mixed-in protein. We want the mineral-protein combination to remain free of positive or negative ions. Otherwise, the mineral will bond with something else and may not be utilized. Note: It is for this reason we suggest that you do not use "Colloidal Minerals!

A mineral plays three roles in the human body:

- It supports the energy conversion process
- It aids in the growth and maintenance of the body's tissues
- They assist in the regulation of all bodily processes.

19

Contrary to popular belief, chelation does not insure absorption of minerals, as this is best achieved by taking mineral supplements with food containing minerals.

The ingestion of fresh food is always the best way to achieve maximum nutrient intake. Individual biochemistry, including enzymatic functions, will generally determine a person's ability to effectively process minerals. However, minerals tied to salts have little bioavailability compared to amino acid chelation.

There are 17 minerals, which humans need. The following nine minerals (out of the seventeen) are essential; insofar, as they are not found in our food supply: boron, iron, magnesium, zinc, selenium, copper, manganese, chromium, and potassium. A good mineral supplement should contain the above nine essential minerals, plus calcium, and phosphorus.

If the supplement lists all of the minerals in equal doses, opt for another choice, as minerals do not occur in nature in equal amounts. Do not rely on a supplement to supply you with all the minerals you need.

Eat fresh vegetables and fruit, beans, fish, turkey and chicken and take a well-formulated vitamin/mineral supplement with fresh food.

Timed-Released

It is better not to use timed-released vitamins. There are exceptions, of course, but they are rare. When it comes to absorption, timed-released nutrients are inferior. Timed-released vitamins are a nice concept, but research shows conclusively that with a timed-released vitamin, the percent of

20

dosage absorbed is low compared to that of a regular non timed-released vitamin. This is especially true of Vitamin-C.

Synergists

Certain vitamins taken without their synergistic sisters are better off not taken at all. No one nutrient occurs in nature all by itself. When Vitamin-C is present in fruit, its sister, the bioflavonoids, always accompanies it. This is extremely important! Minerals occur in nature in certain ratios to each other and they work synergistically, as do the B-vitamins. A good example is cystine. Do not take supplemental cystine without taking at least 3-times as much Vitamin-C as cystine. Taking large amounts of cystine without Vitamin-C can cause cystine stones in the kidneys and urinary bladder. Well made vitamin and mineral supplements are an excellent adjunct to food, but be an informed and aware consumer when choosing your supplements. As you read this book, you will be given valuable information, which is necessary to live a good quality of life. Remember balance and moderation is important too.

Chapter 3 - Sleep and Life Expectancy

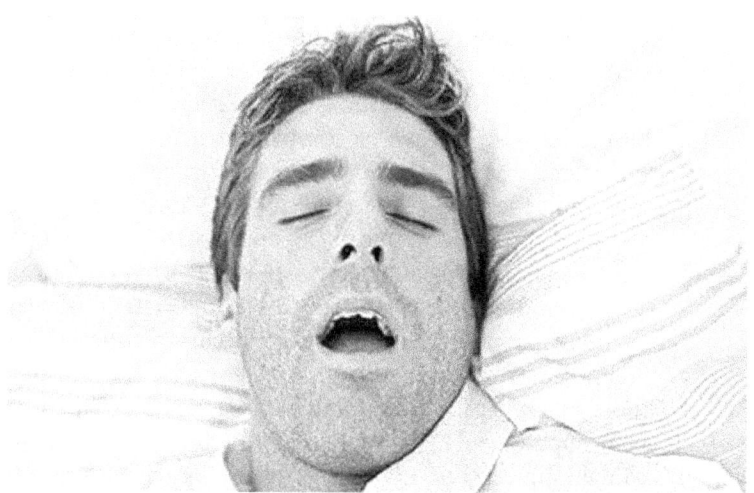

Sleep is getting pretty messed up in modern life. There just doesn't seem to be enough time in the day anymore to get 7 to 9 hours of sleep every day. Can these changes in sleep habits impact life expectancy? That was the question that researchers examined using a large database in the UK.

In a study of 10,308 civil servants in Britain aged 35 to 55, researchers were able to look for links between sleep time and causes of death for more than a 12-year period.

What they found was that decreasing or increasing your sleep time was linked to an increased risk of death. Basically, people who moved out of the 7 to 9 hours of recommended sleep (either less than 7 or more than 9) were more likely to die over the course of the study.

This doesn't mean that sleep itself is to blame. Big shifts in sleep time are common in the case of illnesses, depression and other health conditions.

In fact, medications to treat conditions can cause shifts in sleep time. It could be that sleep time is a marker for overall health. If sleep changes rapidly, it could be a sign that there is a major change in health.

If you find your sleep schedule shifting dramatically, talk to a doctor. You may have a health condition that needs treatment.

Can your sleep habits impact your longevity?

Research has shown that if you sleep too much or not enough, your risk of death increases significantly.

This could be a result of the impact of sleep itself on overall health or it could be because other diseases impact both longevity and sleep duration.

Sleep Duration and Mortality - The Study

In one study, researchers followed over 21,000 twins for more than 22 years. They asked questions about the twins' sleep habits and looked at their longevity. Twins make great research subjects because most of them grew up in the same environment and the have the same (or similar) genetic make-ups. This way researchers can isolate the impact of a behavior (say, sleep duration) to an outcome (like longevity). However, in this study, researchers decided to pool the twin data together - this lost some of the benefit of using twins as a study group. It is not clear why they did this, probably something to do with the way the data was collected.

The participants were asked questions at the beginning of the study and 22 years later. The questions concerned sleep duration, use of sleep medications, and quality of sleep. Researchers were also able to collect data on each participant about their longevity.

The Results - Sleep Duration Linked to Longevity

What the researchers found was that if people slept less than 7 hours a night or more than 8 hours a night, they had an increased risk of

23

death. For short sleep women, that increase was 21% (men: 26%) and for long sleeping women, the increase was 17% (men: 24%). If the participants reported using sleep medications, their risk for death also increased. Women using them had a 39% increase in risk while men had a 31% increase.

Over the course of the study, 30% of the participants changed their sleep habits. The most common change was to shift from stable sleep to short or long sleep. These shifts were also linked to increased risk of mortality.

But What Does It Mean?

The increased risk for different sleep durations may be a cause of more or less sleep, but it may also be true that an underlying factor could cause both changes in sleep and changes in risk. For example, if someone had heart disease, that illness could change how someone sleeps as well as change their risk for death. In short, sleep is at least an indicator (there are others too) of overall health. Changes in sleep or unexplained short/long sleep duration should be taken seriously.

Sleep Deprivation and Heart Disease

I have heard that not getting enough sleep can cause heart disease. Is this true?
Several recent studies have made an association between chronic sleep deprivation (in general, getting fewer than five hours of sleep per night) and heart disease - or at least the risk factors for heart disease.

Short sleep durations have been associated with the development of hypertension, with coronary artery calcification, and with worse outcomes in patients with cardiovascular disease.

Notably, however, one study suggests that not only is fewer than five hours of sleep associated with increased cardiovascular disease, but so is getting too much sleep! That is, people who reported sleeping for more than eight or nine hours per night also had an increased risk of coronary artery disease, stroke or death from cardiovascular causes.

If this latter study is correct, then there is an "optimal sleep range" of roughly between six and eight hours of sleep per night.

There are several theories as to why chronic sleep deprivation may predispose a person to heart disease. Chief among these is that a lack of sleep interferes with certain hormone levels - in particular, leptin and ghrelin - which affect appetite levels and energy expenditure. So, short sleep duration can increase your chances of becoming overweight, sedentary, and developing insulin resistance and metabolic syndrome.

Why too much sleep might be associated with the development of heart disease is completely unknown. It might be that people who have certain medical conditions that predispose to heart disease (such as chronic depression) might also simply sleep more hours.

Your best bet is to try to get a solid six or seven hours of sleep most nights. However, occasionally staying up late (or occasionally sleeping in!) is not particularly hazardous to your health, and in any case is a natural feature of the human condition.

Chapter 4 - Longevity and Illness

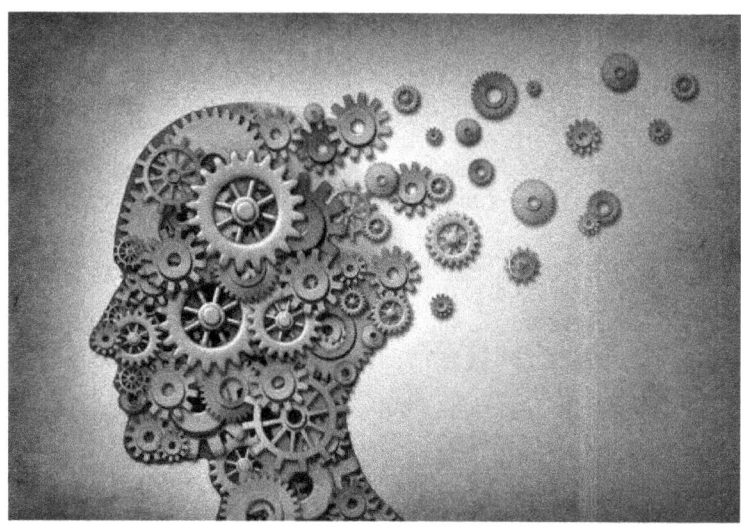

Your Heart and Aging

The heart is an amazing muscle that beats around **100,000 times** a day. It is essentially a complex pump that is able to adjust blood pressure, flow, and volume in order to provide your body with all the blood it needs. Your heart is constantly adjusting to what you are doing and the state of your body. As you age, your heart adjusts to the needs of an older body. These adjustments come with trade-offs, leaving the heart more vulnerable to disease and other problems.

Your Heart's Job:

Everyday your heart must beat more than 100,000 times to pump **1,800 gallons** of blood through more than **60,000 miles** (if stretched end-to-end) of blood vessels. Your heart also must adjust the rate and force at which it pumps based on your activity level. As we age, changes in the body require that the heart adjusts how it works. For example, the buildup of fat in the arteries, known as atherosclerosis, causes the heart to work harder to pump all that blood through narrower tubes.

The Aging Heart:

Heart disease is a leading cause of death. As we age, our heart compensates for clogged arteries by working harder and raising blood pressure. These changes put the heart at risk and impact our quality of life:

- 40 percent of deaths for people aged 65 to 74 are from heart disease (60 percent for those over 80).
- From age 20 to 80, there is a 50 percent decline in the body's capacity for vigorous exercise
- In your 20s the maximum heart is between 180 and 200 beats per minute. At 80, it is 145.
- A 20-year-old's heart can output 3.5 to 4 times the heart's resting capacity. An 80-year-old can output 2 times resting capacity.

Aging Arteries:

Arteries take oxygen-rich blood away from the heart and deliver it to the body. As we age, our arteries become stiffer and less flexible. This causes our blood pressure to increase. The heart has to adjust to the increase in blood pressure by pumping harder and changing the timing of its valves. These adjustments leave the heart more vulnerable. To stay young at heart, protect your arteries by:

- exercising
- controlling your blood pressure
- watching your cholesterol

Thickening of the Left Ventricle:

Researchers have noted that the wall of the left ventricle of the heart becomes thicker with age. This thickening allows the heart to pump stronger. As our blood vessels age, they become narrower -- causing blood pressure to increase. The heart compensates for this by becoming stronger and pumping with more force.

Mitral Valve Closes More Slowly:
The mitral valve closes more slowly with aging. This is because the rate of blood flow from the left ventricle decreases as it relaxes more slowly. It relaxes slower because it grows thicker with age (see above).

Exercise Capacity Shrinks:
As the heart ages, it becomes less able to respond rapidly to chemical messages from the brain. Researchers do not know exactly why the heart does not respond as fast to messages to speed up and adjust to increased activity.

The result is the body cannot exercise as long or as intensely as before. This shows up as shortness of breath -- a sign that oxygen-rich blood is not moving fast enough through the body because the lungs are trying to breath in more oxygen.

"Sitting" Heart Rate Lowers:
The heart rate of an older person while sitting is slower than a younger person (but the same when lying down). It is thought that this slower rate is from a decline in the heart-brain communication because fibrous tissue and fatty deposits have built up on the on nerves connecting the heart and brain. To compensate, the heart increases the volume of blood in circulation by raising the diastolic blood pressure.

The Heart Can't Squeeze as Tightly:

Because of the increase in diastolic blood pressure, the heart also stretches larger each beat, giving a stronger pump in order to have a stronger contraction to pump the excess blood volume (called the Frank-Starling mechanism). But because of the greater diastolic pressure, the heart can't squeeze as tightly.

Heart Enlarges:

The heart of a healthy 70-year-old has 30 percent fewer cells than a 20-year-old's heart. When heart cells die, the other cells must stretch and grow to stay connected. An older person's heart cells may be up to 40 percent larger than younger persons.

Keep Your Heart Healthy and Reverse Heart Disease

Your heart is only as healthy as your arteries. Work hard to keep your arteries healthy by:

- controlling your blood pressure
- improving your cholesterol
- exercising
- relaxing
- learning heart healthy nutrition

Exercise to Prevent Stroke

Your physical health greatly affects your stroke risk. People between the ages of 40 to 79 who can do basic physical tasks may have half the risk of stroke as those who cannot. This is after other health conditions are taken into account (according to a study published in *Neurology*).

How to Improve Physical Functioning

First off, you'll need to start exercising. Your current health status will determine your starting point. After getting cleared by your doctor, find yourself a qualified personal trainer who can help design a program for you. If you can't afford a trainer, find a relative, friend or family member who can help make sure you are doing the exercises correctly.

Then you have to do it. You should have some form of physical activity every day with focused cardio, strength, flexibility and balance weekly. Some great starting points include walking, biking and group classes like yoga. See below for more detail on the study:

Physical Health and Stroke Risk

The study looked at data from 13,615 men and women in the UK from 1993 to 1997 and followed them for 18 months. Over that time, 244 strokes were reported from the group. Using a well-established survey, researchers asked each participant about his physical health. The better a person did on the physical health questions, the less his risk of stroke.

Researchers are not sure the exact way that physical health impacts stroke risk. The researchers believe that poor physical functioning might be a sign of another health condition such as chronic inflammation which could increase stroke risk. They suggest using physical health surveys to help determine who is in need of stroke prevention.

Transfats and Heart Disease

Transfats are created in food processing through the hydrogenation of oils. In short, transfats are artificial and the body has a hard time regulating them. Instead of being digested normally these fats end up in the blood stream as cholesterol. Eventually this leads to atherosclerosis and heart disease. All foods sold in the US must include the amount of transfats on the label. As a simple rule, don't eat any.

Top Ways to Live Longer With Heart Disease

So you have been diagnosed with heart disease, high cholesterol, high blood pressure or some other form of cardiovascular illness. Heart problems often emerge as your heart adjusts to aging. The good news? You can do a lot to control and sometimes reverse these conditions by making lifestyle changes in your life. These changes will not only help your condition, but they'll give you more energy, make you feel better and help you live longer. Go through these 10 items one at a time. When you master one, move onto another that interests you. When you are done with the list, you likely will be healthier.

Hire a Personal Trainer

Your heart is a muscle and it needs its exercise, or it will grow soft and flabby. Getting started in exercise -- especially if you aren't at your peak form right now -- can be mentally and physically challenging.

First, talk with your doctor and get specific guidelines for how much exercise you should do, and how to recognize the signs of overexertion.

Next, find a gym that has personal trainers. The trainer can help make sure that your efforts are going to pay off, and that you are doing the exercises correctly.

Give yourself the best chance you can at jump-starting an exercise program -- hire a trainer.

Hire a Nutritionist/Dietitian

You will probably only need 1 or 2 consultations with a nutritionist to learn volumes about what you are eating, what you should be eating, and why. To get the most out of your consultation, bring 2 or 3 days of food logs with you.

A food log is simply a record of everything you eat or drink in a day, the times you ate or drank it, and the amounts. This will help the nutritionist tailor a program to your life.

Banish your Enemies

You have food enemies -- you know what they are: cookies, ice cream, chips or maybe candy.

- You must banish these from your house, from your car, from your office.
- You can no longer purchase these items.
- You can no longer eat them on a regular basis.

If they show up at a party or special occasion you can have some -- but you can no longer buy or seek them out. Ever!

Relax a Little

Stress constricts your blood vessels, and this makes it harder for your heart to pump blood through your body. Relax. Let the events of the day wash over you. Learn relaxation breathing. Try to keep the big picture in mind -- ask yourself, will the stress triggers matter five years from now? Will you even remember them?

Smile

Smiling does all sorts of good for your body. You can actually trick your body and mind into being happy by smiling. Put a smile on your face while

- standing in line
- while driving
- while writing e-mails

You'll be amazed at the change. Practice by smiling every time you look at a clock. This will add hundreds of smiles to your day.

Learn to Cook

Have you ever been amazed by restaurants? You can walk in; order any one of 70 items off a menu and a few minutes later your meal arrives warm and delicious. It is like a miracle. And the name of that miracle is **butter**. Restaurants use fats and butter to cover up so-so ingredients, over warming and other sins of necessity. By learning to cook and eating at home, you can be in control of your food. Use fresh ingredients and take some cooking classes.

Monitor and Record

- Monitor your blood pressure weekly; keep your test results in a folder for easy access.
- Have your cholesterol tested every few months.
- Keep track of your medical information.
- Know what medications you are on, who your doctors are and what your medical goals are.

By keeping all this information at your fingertips, you can help your doctor(s) plan the best medical care for you.

Take Your Medicine

If you doctor has prescribed medicine for you, take it. Figure out what you need to do to take your medicine at the right times and following the suggestions.

There are some really excellent medications on the market now that have helped millions of people avoid heart attacks and other problems. Be **100 percent compliant** with your doctor's orders.

Invest in People

People with health conditions do better if they have strong social relationships. Your spouse, friend, or family member can be there to

- help you overcome challenges
- make lifestyle changes
- And assist you if you are ill.

It has also been shown that having close relationships will also help you reduce stress and improve healing. So take a second honeymoon, go on a buddy fishing trip, or have a spa day with someone you care about.

Celebrate Life

Life is good. Celebrate the progress you make in creating a healthier you.

- Celebrate your success, the people around you.
- Seek out and enjoy wonderful things.

- Don't get caught in routines and ruts that eat away your days.
- Plan to celebrate something every week -- go to art museums, symphonies, and jazz bars.
- Build something.
- Paint, draw, play.

Chapter 5 - Low-Carb and Diabetes

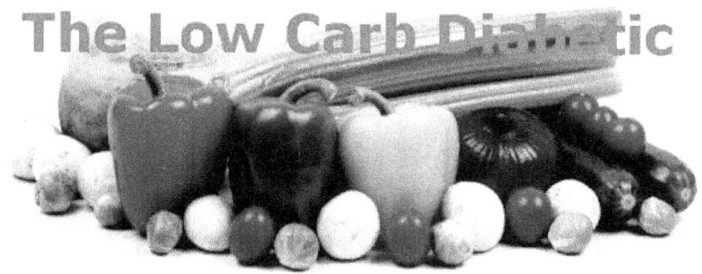

The diet recommended by the American Diabetes Association (ADA) contains moderate levels of carbohydrates. Some in the diabetes field wonder if restricting carbohydrate consumption further might even reverse diabetes.

Men's Health magazine reported that the ADA diet was primarily constructed to reduce a diabetic's risk of heart disease, which is the number one killer of diabetics. Therapeutic nutrition for diabetes is an unexplored area. Individuals at risk for developing diabetes could benefit by reducing simple carbohydrate consumption and should consult a nutritionist.

Three Ways to Reduce Cholesterol

Cholesterol is an important thing to monitor and reduce when it comes to longevity. High cholesterol means (simply) that your body has too much gunk in your arteries. That gunk can lead to heart attacks and stroke. It's a good thing that lowering your cholesterol through lifestyle changes and medication is possible. Follow these three simple steps to increase your longevity and live longer. Reward yourself then with these fun ways to live longer.

Change Your Diet

Reduce the amount of fat that you eat in your diet. Avoid fatty meats, cheeses, and processed foods (especially fast food). You can do this simply by increasing the amount of vegetables and treating meat as a side dish. Avoid all the obvious fatty foods (like ice cream) and focus on eating lots and lots of fruits and vegetables.

Exercise

Exercise helps the body break down cholesterol. Work up a sweat at least three times a week for at least 30 minutes each time. You can do anything you want to work up a sweat - you don't have to go to the gym. Try speed walking, stair climbing or good old-fashioned jumping jacks.

Take Your Medication

There are a number of good anti-cholesterol medications. Ask your doctor about them, but always make lifestyle changes too -- your goal should be to live healthy and eventually not need the medication. And remember to take your medicine after you get it. A shocking number of people don't take medicine that could save your life. Work your medicine into your daily routine and don't skip any doses.

Chapter 6 - Alzheimer's Disease and Life Expectancy

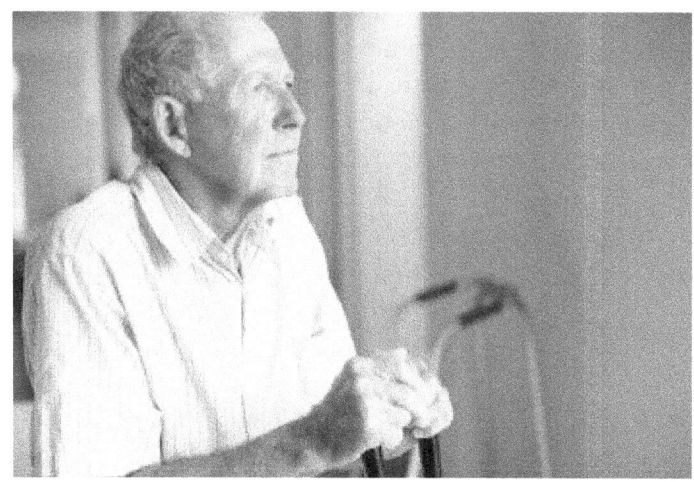

Alzheimer's disease and other illness involving dementia are considered understudied. There are 24 million people in the world with Alzheimer's disease or other forms of dementia, and this number is growing rapidly. This number is expected to triple to 81 million by 2040.

Alzheimer's Disease, Dementia and Life Expectancy

Researchers followed 13,000 people over the age of 65 from 1991 to 2005 to better understand diseases of dementia. Over that time, 438 people in the study developed Alzheimer's disease or another form of dementia. 81% of those developing dementia died before the study was completed.

Age and Gender Main Factors for Alzheimer's Disease and Dementia Longevity

The main factors that determined how long a person in the study lived after being diagnosed with Alzheimer's disease or another form of dementia were age, gender and level of disability. Here are the main findings:

- Women lived an average of 4.6 years after diagnosis, men lived 4.1 years.
- People diagnosed when under age 70 lived 10.7 years compared to 3.8 years for people over 90 when diagnosed.
- Patients who were frail at the time of diagnosis did not live as long, even after adjusting for age.
- Overall, the average survival time for someone in the study diagnosed with Alzheimer's disease or dementia was 4.5 years.

Why Do Alzheimer's Disease and Dementia Shorten Life?

The average 65-year-old can expect to live 18.5 years longer – almost double the amount after being diagnosed with Alzheimer's disease or dementia. The study did not examine the reasons for this shorter life expectancy. In the group that was diagnosed after age 90, one would expect shorter life expectancies simply due to their advanced age. The loss of life expectancy in the younger group could be attributed to lifestyle changes caused by dementia such as no longer exercising or eating well, but that doesn't explain everything. It could also be that early onset Alzheimer's disease and dementia take a different course than the later onset types. So, from the research, we know the average life expectancies, but we don't know why.

How To Help Someone With Dementia

While you can't change factors such as age at diagnosis or gender, the study did show that the level of care that a person receives impacts life expectancy. Be sure that you explore options when it comes to creating a care plan for a loved one diagnosed with Alzheimer's disease and take advantage of any support groups or other resources that may help.

Preventing Alzheimer's Disease and Dementia

There have been many studies looking into the use of puzzles and other forms of "mental fitness" to help delay or prevent Alzheimer's disease and dementia. A famous study of nuns showed that the individuals most curious and engaged mentally in the world had less Alzheimer's disease and dementia.

Chapter 7 - Live Longer with Prostate Cancer

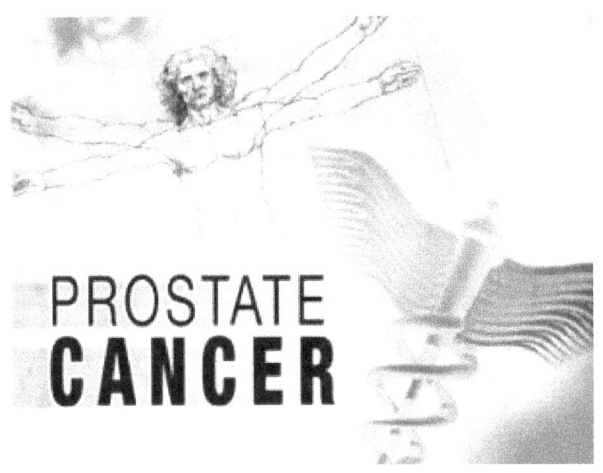

Prostate cancer treatments cover a wide range of approaches that impact life expectancy differently. Believe it or not, no formal clinical studies have been done to determine how best to treat localized prostate cancer. These studies would be extremely difficult to do - - they would take up to 10 years to complete, people would have to be randomly assigned to different treatment groups and the cost would be quite high. So instead, researchers have taken data from the past to compare treatments. This is called a retrospective (or historical) study. Keep in mind that there may be factors unknown to the researchers reviewing medical charts that impact the outcome.

Life Expectancy and Localized Prostate Cancer

Swiss researchers examined the treatment and outcomes of 844 patients diagnosed with localized prostate cancer sometime between 1989 and 1998. Five different types of treatment were applied (the "n" indicates the number of participants):

- prostatectomy (surgical removal of the prostate) n=158
- radiotherapy (radiation treatment) n=205
- watchful waiting (monitoring the cancer) n=378
- hormone therapy n=72
- other treatments n=31

Survival and Life Expectancy in Localized Prostate Cancer

The researchers looked at the survival rates for each group and found that at five years from diagnosis, the type of treatment made little difference to survival. When the researchers went to 10 years from diagnosis, they did find a difference in survival based on treatment. Overall, 10-year survival was:

- 83% for prostatectomy
- 75% for radiotherapy
- 72% for watchful waiting

Those who had hormone risk had decreased survival rates at 5 years, but this is almost certainly because their cancer was a much more aggressive type when they were diagnosed.

Is Prostatectomy the Best Treatment for Prostate Cancer Then?

You cannot conclude that from this study. What we don't know is why certain people were given the treatment they received. It could be the Swiss doctors have a preference. For example, they might prefer a prostectomy when the cancer presents a certain way and radiotherapy when it "looks" different. In other words, this study tells us that prostectomy is the most effective OR that doctors tend to send patients with less threatening tumors for prostectomies OR (more likely) a complex combination of both (and throw in some other factors too). Confused yet? Sorry about that. But it is important that you understand the limitations of these studies. Ask your doctor what factors he or she uses to decide on treatment and engage with that discussion.

Reverse Metabolic Syndrome to Live Longer

If you are like most people, you are confused. The news and doctors talk about metabolic syndrome, syndrome X and insulin resistance syndrome. Basically, these are three different terms for the same thing. What they mean is, "heading for trouble."

Metabolic Syndrome, Syndrome X and Insulin Resistance

These three terms are used to describe an increased risk of cardiovascular disease and diabetes. The most common term is metabolic syndrome (I'll use that term from now on). This term describes a condition in which a number of risk factors (like high blood pressure) are combined. The good news is that the increased risk for cardiovascular disease and diabetes can be reversed through aggressive lifestyle changes and (in some cases) medication.

Diagnosing Metabolic Syndrome

Metabolic syndrome is diagnosed using a combination of measurements and blood tests. There are basically five numbers that doctors will check. If three of the five are not in healthy levels, a patient may be diagnosed with metabolic syndrome.

Definition of Metabolic Syndrome

Here are the five things that define metabolic syndrome, if three or more are present then a person is said to have "metabolic syndrome":

1. Waist circumference greater than 40 inches in men or greater than 35 inches in women
2. High blood pressure
3. Elevated fasting blood sugar (more than 110 mg/dL)
4. Elevated triglycerides
5. Low levels of HDL cholesterol (the good cholesterol)

Each of these tests shows signs of trouble. If three or more of these is in the unhealthy range, then that person's risk of stroke, heart attack and diabetes is elevated.

Treatment and Prevention of Metabolic Syndrome

You already know how to treat and prevent metabolic syndrome -- live healthy. Exercise, weight loss and eating a healthy diet can help reverse metabolic syndrome. Your doctor may suggest a combination of lifestyle change and medication, or may give you a "trial" period to give lifestyle change a chance while monitoring you closely. Take this **very** seriously. Make all the changes you possibly can and don't cheat. The good news is that the improvements you make will have you sleeping better and feeling energized.

Chapter 8 - Aging and Eye Diseases

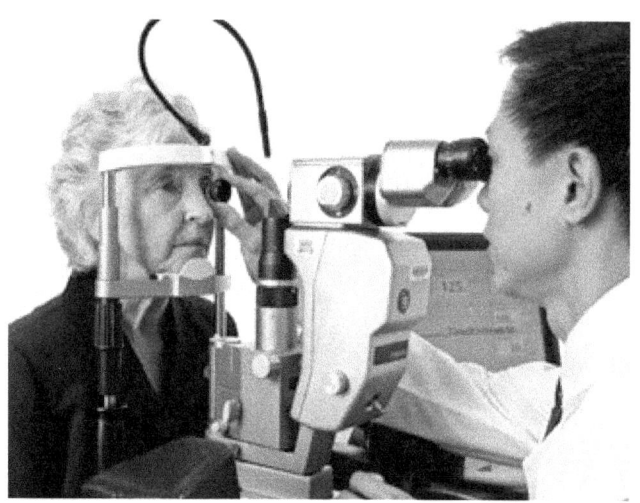

Eye disorders and diseases are common in older adults. Laser surgeries and other treatments exist to correct and even reverse some of these conditions. The key is to detect them early. Regular eye exams will help detect vision problems before they become serious. Here is a list of common age-related eye problems:

Cataracts: Your eye has a lens that helps it to focus. The lens is made of protein. When protein molecules clump, a cloudy spot (called a cataract) forms. This is common in older people. Because cataracts grow slowly, your eye doctor may simply monitor a cataract until it interferes with your vision. Cataract surgery is a very common procedure to remove the cataract from your eye.

Dry Eye: Your eyelids have lacrimal glands that produce tears, and they drain into your tear ducts in your lower eyelids.

If your lacrimal glands stop working well, your eyes will become dry and uncomfortable. Eye drops can help, but have your eyes checked. There may be a simple procedure to partially plug your tear ducts (to keep tears from draining too fast).

Glaucoma: The eye is filled with fluid. If too much pressure develops in the eye, it is called glaucoma. Over time, this build-up of pressure can damage the optic nerve and cause blindness. Luckily, this pressure develops slowly and routine eye exams can detect glaucoma before it becomes dangerous.

Age-Related Macular Degeneration (AMD): This is a very long term for loss of central vision. The macula is a part of the retina that processes central vision. Sometimes with aging, the macula deteriorates. This causes problems with driving, reading and many common tasks. Treatment can include laser surgery on the macula.

Diabetic Retinopathy: Because of problems with diabetes, the tiny blood vessels that supply oxygen and nutrients to the retina become less effective, which leads to vision problems. Treatment includes laser surgery and a surgical process known as a vitrectomy. All diabetics should have annual eye exams.

Retinal Detachment: The layers of the retina can detach from the underlying support tissue. If untreated, retinal detachment can cause loss of vision or blindness. Symptoms include an increase in the type and number of "floaters" in your eyes, seeing bright flashes, feeling as if a curtain has been pulled over the field of vision, or seeing straight lines that appear curvy. Surgery and laser treatment can often reattach the layers of the retina.

Your Vision and Aging

As you age, your eyes change. Certain parts of the eyes become less elastic, which impacts how well you can focus at close range. Cells may clump, causing floaters. These and other changes are a natural part of aging. This is a list of some common vision problems that happen along with aging. This list does not include age-related eye diseases and disorders.

- Reading the Fine Print: The loss of being able to see close objects is a normal part of aging. This is known as presbyopia. It is thought to be caused by a loss of elasticity of the lens of the eye. Simple and inexpensive reading glasses can help.
- Floaters: When you are in a bright room, you may notice little specks that seem to float across your eye. These are actually small clumps of cells in the vitreous fluid that fills the eye. Floaters occur naturally with age and are harmless. If you notice an increase or change in floaters or see floaters along with bright flashes, see an eye doctor promptly.
- Tearing: With age, the eyes become more sensitive to wind and light. You may find yourself tearing very easily. Dry eyes are one cause of increased tearing. To reduce tearing, start by protecting your eyes - wear sunglasses to reduce glare and protect your eyes from the wind. If your tearing becomes a problem, see your eye doctor; you could have a blocked tear duct or other problem.

Vision and Aging Tips

Your vision will change as you age. Whether you need to deal with some loss of vision or are looking for a way to protect your vision, these ten tips can help:

See Your Eye Doctor

See your eye doctor whenever you have a problem with your eyes. You eye doctor can help dry eyes, itchy eyes and excessive tearing. Diabetics need to have an eye exam every year. People over 40 should go at least once every five years.

Eye Drops

If you have dry eyes, eye drops can keep your eyes moist and comfortable. This is important because moist eyes are able to wash out particles, viruses and bacteria that can cause eye infections and irritations.

Don't Smoke

Smoking increases your risk of a number of eye diseases. Avoiding smoking, and quit now if you do smoke. Smoke speeds up the damage to your eye due to the free radicals in tobacco smoke and other factors.

Wash Your Hands and Don't Touch

By washing your hands and not touching your eyes frequently, you can greatly reduce your risk of eye infections. Be sure to wash your hands often during the day and keep them away from your eyes.

Lots of Fruits and Vegetables

Fruits and vegetables provide essential vitamins and antioxidants that keep your eyes healthy. Try to eat a variety of colors of fruits and vegetables every day. Be sure to include some dark-colored ones.

Take a Multivitamin

There are some vitamins that are essential to eye health. To be sure you are getting the right vitamins, take a daily multivitamin. This will help protect your night vision and keep your eyes healthy throughout your life.

Manage Your Health Conditions

High blood pressure, diabetes and other chronic illnesses can impact the health of your eyes. By making the necessary lifestyle changes and managing your illness according to your doctor's guidance, you can avoid some of the eye-related complications of many chronic illnesses.

Use Contrast

If you notice that you are having trouble seeing, try to add contrast to poorly lit places. Putting a dark piece of tape on a lightly colored step can make a big difference in judging the step accurately. Increasing the difference between light and dark colors in your home can help you avoid falls and continue to function normally.

Better Lighting

Lighting can impact your ability to see. Use bright, full-spectrum lights whenever possible. Change your light bulbs and be sure that you have enough light to see clearly. If you notice vision problems, better lighting can help tremendously.

Sunglasses

Sunglasses are not just a fashion accessory; they protect your eyes in three ways:

- They filter out harmful UV rays
- They keep dirt and other particles away from your eyes
- They keep your eyes from drying out due to wind

These three benefits will help keep your eyes feeling comfortable and prevent irritation and infection.

Chapter 9 - Your Hearing and Aging

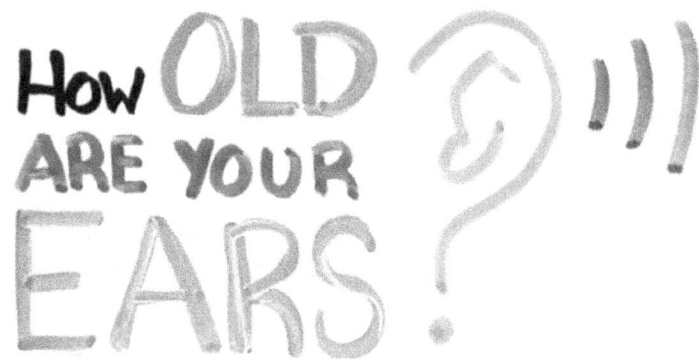

Age-related hearing loss, also called presbycusis, is the gradual loss of the ability to hear sounds (often high-pitched sounds). This loss of ability occurs so slowly that many people are not aware that they have hearing loss.

Causes of Age-Related Hearing Loss

The most common cause of hearing loss in aging adults is a loss of tiny hair cells in the ear. These cells act as receptors – they vibrate when sounds are present. The loss of hair cells is largely thought to be due to aging itself, though the following factors may also be important in some cases:

- The combined effect of a lifetime of exposure to loud noises, such as traffic, construction work, noisy offices, heavy machinery, and loud music.
- Hereditary factors – people who have family members with hearing loss are more likely to have hearing loss as they age.

- Some health conditions, like heart disease, high blood pressure, and diabetes, can cause presbycusis because they affect the blood supply available to the ear.
- Some medications, such as aspirin and certain antibiotics, have also been found to contribute to presbycusis.

Symptoms

For a person with presbycusis, sounds seem deeper and less clear. Other symptoms can include:

- Others' speech seems mumbled or slurred
- High-pitched sounds are difficult to hear
- Conversations are hard to follow
- Background noise interferes with hearing
- Men's voices are easier to hear than women's
- Ringing in the ears (tinnitus)

Treatment

Some people with presbycusis may need hearing aids. Hearing aids and other assistive hearing devices can help in certain situations, such as using a telephone. There are modifications that a person can make to his or her environment to help with hearing.

Prevention

Hearing loss caused by exposure to loud noises can be prevented. Become aware of loud noises in your environment and take action to prevent them from damaging your ears. Earplugs should be used when you are exposed to firearms, lawn mowers, leaf blowers, jet skies, power tools, loud appliances, and snowmobiles. Be sure to keep the volume moderate when using headphones, and always wear earplugs at concerts.

The Stats

About 30 to 35 percent of people between the ages of 65 and 75 have some form of hearing loss. This can include partial hearing loss, the inability to hear certain frequencies, or hearing loss in one ear. Almost 50 percent of people over the age of 75 have some form of hearing loss with 30 percent of those over the age 85 having deafness in at least one ear.

Hearing Loss Tips

These tips can help improve communication with people with hearing loss. If you know someone who has trouble listening, practice these tips. If you have hearing loss, ask the people you talk with most to follow these suggestions:

- Talk while facing the person.
- Don't speak too fast.
- Don't mumble.
- Don't hide your mouth, chew gum, or eat while speaking.
- Be expressive--hand gestures and facial expressions can help give clues about what you're saying.
- If asked to repeat yourself, try using different words than the first time.
- Reduce or eliminate background noises, like a radio or television.
- Don't speak for or answer for a hearing impaired person when talking with others. Give him or her time to respond.
- Don't shout – it distorts your words.

- Relax, be patient, and have a good sense of humor.
- Ask how else you can help.

I Have a Special Gift for My Readers

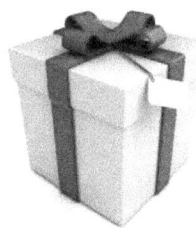

I appreciate my readers for without them I am just another author attempting to make a difference. If my book has made a favorable impression please leave me an honest review. Thank you in advance for you participation.

My readers and I have in common a passion for the written word as well as the desire to learn and grow from books.

My special offer to you is a massive ebook library that I have compiled over the years. It contains hundreds of fiction and non-fiction ebooks in Adobe Acrobat PDF format as well as the Greek classics and old literary classics too.

In fact, this library is so massive to completely download the entire library will require over 5 GBs open on your desktop.

Use the link below and scan all of the ebooks in the library. You can select the ebooks you want individually or download the entire library.

The link below does not expire after a given time period so you are free to return for more books rather than clog your desktop. And feel free to give the link to your friends who enjoy reading too.

I thank you for reading my book and hope if you are pleased that you will leave me an honest review so that I can improve my work and or write books that appeal to your interests.

Okay, here is the link…

http://tinyurl.com/special-readers-promo

PS: If you wish to reach me personally for any reason you may simply write to mailto:support@epubwealth.com.

I answer all of my emails so rest assured I will respond.

Meet the Author

Dr. Noah Pranksky is a research behavioral scientist for Applied Mind Sciences. His research involves many aspects of the human mind including relationships, energy psychology, and various protocols and modalities relating to treatment and cure of various mental maladies.

He and his wife Marianne reside in Portland, Oregon.

Visit some of his websites
http://www.AddMeInNow.com
http://www.AppliedMindSciences.com
http://www.AppliedWebInfo.com
http://www.BookbuilderPLUS.com
http://www.BookJumping.com
http://www.EmailNations.com
http://www.EmbarrassingProblemsFix.com
http://www.ePubWealth.com
http://www.ForensicsNation.com
http://www.ForensicsNationStore.com

http://www.FreebiesNation.com
http://www.HealthFitnessWellnessNation.com
http://www.Neternatives.com
http://www.PrivacyNations.com
http://www.RetireWithoutMoney.org
http://www.SurvivalNations.com
http://www.TheBentonKitchen.com
http://www.Theolegions.org
http://www.VideoBookbuilder.com